On Organic Living

Life Hacks for the Eco-Conscious Soul

Please visit the Organic Publishing House website at:

www.organicpublishinghouse.org

And

Flora Jade's website at:

www.theflorajade.com

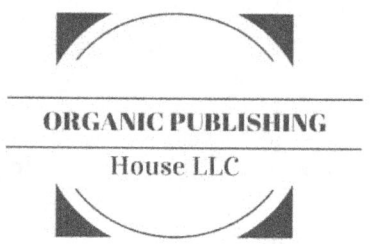

Organic Publishing House LLC

· Seattle ·

CONTENTS

On Organic Living

Life Hacks for the Eco-Conscious Soul

Flora Jade

To my family.

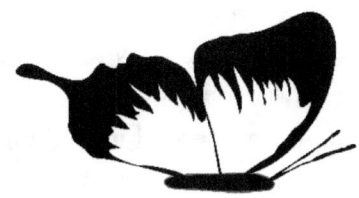

Introduction: Organic Living

$\mathscr{F}$or beginning or supplementing your organic minded life, this book is a compilation of simple tips and tricks from over fifteen years of organic living. Generations prior normally had fewer options and used more chemicals than in this day and age. Because we are now more aware than ever of the world around us in all facets, we can research most ingredients in products we bring inside the home. As many harsh chemicals have been revealed to have serious health implications, we see the benefit of going green or natural. Still, even though "natural" has little bearing on organic goods, since everything is by some definition natural, we'll use it as a way to describe products that are less chemically infused and are petroleum free. Another example of recent important knowledge we have that our forebears did not is how superbugs could evolve from our super cleaner use. The more we learn, the safer our world can become.

Many natural options to avoid these harsh chemicals are found throughout the book in an array of inexpensive, natural, and homemade alternatives to brand-name organic products. Some surprising and misrepresented ingredients—found in common products we use, consume, and wear—are concerning, and will be discussed throughout. Like the farm to table movement with food, we need to go back to our roots and reevaluate what passes over the threshold of our home.

This book is for all levels of people's experiences in organic living practices, covering many categories with concessions so you don't always have to buy organic, as it can be hard on the pocket book. Organic-minded shopping can be made less strict. The goal in mind is to make organic buying stress free by being easy to follow. Only a few organically minded shopping trips will enable us to target important products. (Please note that the sources for information in this book may be found at the end of the volume—Ed.)

Everyone can ultimately discover their need and the rewards for a change toward a more organic life. People make the move for many reasons such as general sensitivity to chemicals, allergies to an additive in foods, stomach pangs from over use of antibacterial products, pet or family member allergies to detergents, or concerns about useful yet dangerous chemicals in our homes. No matter the reason for your increasing awareness and appreciation of natural and organic living, there's no better time to start than now. By incorporating gradual changes in the way you view your home, you can build your sanctuary for peaceful livelihoods and a productive, healthy family.

Organic Food Tips

"Let food be thy medicine and medicine thy food."

—Hippocrates

$\mathscr{S}$etting up a family home conducive to healthy living and to a thriving family begins in the kitchen. Whether you've already made the switch to incorporating organic foods and products in your life, or are ready to begin, you have your story as to why you decided to make the change. For many, the switch is made because of concerns over their child's exposure to pesticides and insecticides, the impact of chemicals on fertility in women, a bewildering variety of digestion issues, or even worries about the presence of known or potential carcinogenic properties of commonly used products. The reasons to make the change to organic are countless.

Some people may resist switching to organic because of cost, but the number of products with minimal markup is growing as demand increases. No longer do we have to drive an extra 15 minutes out of the way to find organic milk or produce, only to have it expire within two days of purchase. These days organic inventory turns over faster as more people switch to organic groceries. For the ultimate benefits to our health, spending a dollar more here or there on organic foods might be worth trying. Finding budget-friendly organic foods and dairy products is easier than ever.

Start by stocking a kitchen that is organic and free of genetically modified organisms (GMO). Then, simply by using the recipe building blocks you will find here, you can begin to prepare safer and more nutritious meals.

These are the must-have organic items to begin with because they tend to be the most heavily treated with chemicals in standard, non-organic production for general food markets. Replacing them in your daily food regimen would be a major start for a program of health through organics, especially because organic versions have become increasingly available:

Apples
Berries
Carrots
Celery

Cherries
Corn Meal • Corn Flour • Grits
Dairy
Flour
Grapes
Lettuce (greens)
Meat
Nuts
Peppers
Poultry
Potatoes
Seeds
Soy Products (Soy alternatives for meat • Soymilk •
Soybeans • Soybean Oil • Tofu)
Stone Fruit
Tomatoes

The simple trick to buying organic is, *if you can eat the skin, buy organic*; *if not, buy standard.* An example of this is almonds. While you don't eat the skin, they do grow inside of an apricot-like stone fruit and should be an organic purchase. Another example is avocado, which you can buy standard. Most of the other pantry and kitchen staples are okay to buy standard. If it's in the budget go ahead and buy all organic, but this is a great place to start. Cruciferous vegetables such as broccoli, Brussels sprouts, and cabbage are self-insect repelling and are generally okay to buy standard. Many countries have fully regulated organic farms but take that with a grain of salt. Some countries value production volume, and therefore income, over standards of quality. Check the country of origin as the farms in many countries outside of the United States (US) have differing organic standards and their food products might be laced with chemicals that are banned here. Some countries, especially in Europe, routinely market organic produce, even without labeling them so. When in doubt about imports, take a trip to the local farmers' market and support your area's local organic farmers.

Shopping local and organic eliminates the risk of GMOs. At least in the US, GMO crops are not allowed to have the organic label. While not all GMOs are bad, the worst offenders are engineered to naturally resist herbicides. This enables GMO farmers to spray crops heavily with herbicides and insecticides without risk of killing the crop itself. Massive amounts of these chemicals end up on our dinner table. For instance, the majority of soybeans grown in the US have been genetically modified so it's best to go organic or find the most natural brands. Corn grown for milling is also engineered and is thus a heavily sprayed crop.

Now that even weeds are evolving immunities to herbicides, it's become even more crucial that soil and food production take a more environmentally conscious approach. The cancer risks of exposure to herbicides and pesticides are a major consequence. The cross-pollinating of GMO crops into neighboring standard fields is a concern for farmers wanting only natural and organic crops in their fields. Concerns about herbicides in waterways supplying and therefore contaminating standard crops are especially prominent. Luckily, sweet corn and popcorn are never GMO because GMO corn doesn't contain enough moisture to pop properly, and sweet corn grows well without needing to be sprayed.

Environmental contamination is also a problem in the production of strawberries. Avoid all strawberries (yes, anything organic, too) as the Food and Drug Administration (FDA) allows highly toxic chemicals to be applied to the soil before planting. Large production farmers will continue methyl bromide treatment on strawberry fields as a fumigation technique. In 2017, this chemical treatment will be banned due to its toxicity. Organic strawberry starter plants are typically standard grown and are a lesser-known oversight of the industry. Eco-friendly grown strawberries or wild strawberries are always an option if available at your local farmers' market.

There are also endangering production loopholes in the processing of organic chicken. As of 2013, the federal government has allowed export of live animals to China for processing before returning the meat and byproducts to the US for sale. This potentially inhumane transportation doesn't require regulation in processing in China and is a general food safety concern. Keep this in mind when purchasing from large producers of chicken. As of late 2015, meats for sale in the US under the previous Country of Origin Labeling law no longer have to be labeled with the country of origin. There is an exception for chicken and lamb, which still need labels showing their origin. In the next chapter, we will address additional grave issues surrounding labeling. Support local butchers and local farmers by buying from trustworthy nearby sources.

To preserve the health of the world's wildlife and rainforests, avoid products with palm oil. This culinary oil is a result of the nonsustainable slashing and burning of rainforests, which completely destroys the living environments on which the survival of orangutans and other sensitive species depend. Many companies substitute palm oil for butter, so standard purchases like peel-and-pop dough in tubes, popcorn, and other snacks utilize this endangering oil source. Palm oil can be difficult to avoid at first but as you make the switch to organic foods, know that it isn't generally used in them.

Now that major pesticides are known by the EPA to be detrimental to mammals and overall ecology, it's imperative to increase testing and even ban such chemicals. These chemicals work their way into the immediate environment, which includes our residential water sources for drinking and bathing, but also in many building materials of our homes. Organic pesticides are the more natural alternative, and the physical pulling of weeds is a healthful alternative to the application of broad-spectrum herbicides. Allowing chickens and ducks to roam free will help control pests. These fowl use their natural instincts to eradicate insect crop destroyers. This throwback technique to farming shines light on the inherent value of some time-tested farming practices.

European foods have higher standards in production. Many of the insecticides and herbicides that are allowed in the US are banned in Europe. Their food is considered organic by US standards and is friendly to the environment. Knowing that entire countries take a more practical and healthful approach to food production bodes well for the future of the organic food movement in the US. Later in the chapter we'll compare other food practices between Europe and the US.

In Any Amount: It's Too Much

Food accumulates potential toxins from the earth, but could also be contaminated by contact with storage containers and preparation tools. These interactions can leach toxins or heavy metals into any food or beverage with prolonged contact or heat from microwaves or cooking utensils. Making food preparation choices so we don't ingest such toxins is another method to living naturally.

Phthalates are found in plastics and other petroleum-based products that can work their way into food. This toxic chemical is an ester used in the production of plastics and other products as a thickening agent. Bisphenol A (BPA) and bisphenol S (BPS) are both specific phthalates in plastics. BPS is the new king of plastics now that BPA has been discovered to cause adverse effects in the endocrine system. This chapter shares some tips to eliminate or reduce exposure to plastics and other petroleum-based products.

Manufacturers of canned foods are slowly introducing BPA-free liners in the more health conscious brands that know the effects of BPA and plastics on the body. BPA is a phthalate with the potential, like others in its class, to interfere with normal hormone levels in the human body. Coatings containing BPA commonly line soda cans, food cans, and lids of glass bottles, thus causing BPA to leach into the products being contained. Plastic coatings also have several harmful chemicals besides BPA so it's generally advisable to avoid canned foods, as well. Excessive BPA ingestion is linked to inflammation in the body and heart palpitations. Although neither of the symptoms might outweigh the convenience of canned food for some people, remember that plastics that leach chemicals in the body haven't yet been studied fully. Making a switch and creating your own tomato purée, sauces, beans, and soups—taking the natural approach to any food—adds maximum nutrition without BPA. Homemade food stored in glass storage containers is a go-to meal option. The containers themselves could be sealed with a BPA-free lid and may be used like any other glass bakeware. Further down in the chapter we will discuss more possibilities with glass containers.

Before consuming canned foods or drinks, quickly rinse or wash off the containers before opening, especially if they have not been kept stored in a larger box. Grocery stores continuously move a variety of goods and chemicals around. While efficient, this practice is not necessarily sanitary (pests are found everywhere) nor do they necessarily keep the fertilizer away from the canned goods at all times. Many former or current grocery store employees might suggest you take the time to rinse containers before opening, having direct experience with the contamination potential. Although restaurants are required by health codes to store food and chemicals at a safe distance from each other, storerooms in some grocery stores might not do so in practical operations.

The last place one would expect to be exposed to BPA is while grocery shopping itself. Both you and the cashier are subject to high amounts of BPA in the paper receipts. Heat applied in the printing process of modern receipt machines requires phthalate-coated paper, which is printed without ink. Make sure to place all receipts in an envelope for accounting reasons or recycle them to limit BPA and BPS exposure, particularly because BPA and BPS are harmful to children's endocrine systems and to fertility in women. Because skin, a semi-permeable membrane, is porous, the more receipts that are handled, the more BPA is absorbed by the body. Many department stores are going paperless and will email you the receipt. This is an ideal option as you limit exposure while also saving some trees. If you're worried about spam emails from some companies who opt your email into mass email advertising chains, set up an extra email account for receipts.

It's free and as easy to set up as any other social media account. Also, signing up for an email list often gets you discount coupons which are exclusive to those on the lists.

BPA in conventional disposable plastic water bottles will leach readily into the water when left out in the sun and should be discarded, such as by being sprinkled on the plants outside. People with more sensitive taste buds can taste when water was left in a hot shipping truck or storage room. Concerns over local water supplies in many major cities across the US are an added reason to ensure safe water sources. Buy your water in the colder months and store enough for occasional bottled-water access through the hot summer. Using a reusable glass-lined or stainless steel thermos, glass bottle, or stainless steel coffee cup for your on-the-go water needs is also an easy way to reduce your carbon footprint while limiting or eliminating hazards to the environment and your health.

The quality of the water in your home is often taken for granted, but in light of recent events it's important to learn about any chemicals being added to your water source, as some are especially harmful for you and your family. Worries about heavy metals, toxic chemicals, and pathogens in the municipal water supply are growing in all cities. Filtering your own water or buying aquifer or natural spring water is a way to avoid exposure to unknown contaminants. Knowing the source of any form of bottled water you buy is important because many mass-market soda companies bottle tap water as well. In some parts of the US, ground water is contaminated by fracking as a consequence of this controversial oil harvesting. Be discriminate about drinking or using water near these sources and utilize options for clean water.

Fluoride and chlorine are also a concern. These two elements are especially hard on pets' kidneys as their body mass is lower than in their human owners and might therefore prove toxic in overdose. Remove any possibility of overexposure with high quality gravity filters or water delivery service for dispensers in the home. By ordering large reusable containers of water or consuming safe tap water with these methods, we can achieve peace of mind and maintain the good health of family pets we are responsible for. Giving the entire family access to natural water sources ensures proper hydration without worry. We are made of mostly water so to stay hydrated it's important we bathe in, cook with, and consume clean, mineral rich, and pure water.

When reaching for drinkware, barware, or cookware, first consider their raw material components. Some barware glasses are leaded for clarity. While they may look elegant, they also add the special danger of lead, a heavy metal, to your food and drink. Heavy metals are naturally occurring in the environment and are especially harmful to all life. The toxic nature of certain heavy metals like lead, mercury, and arsenic causes an array of ailments; from cancer to gastric distress and cognitive deficits. They are all extremely difficult for the body to purge after they settle in all organs, especially ones that don't purge toxins easily. Leaded glass may also be known as leaded crystal or simply crystal glassware. *The longer the liquid stays in the glass and the more acidic the beverage, the more lead you can consume.* It's important not to second-guess buying or using leaded glass or crystal by sticking to traditional—unleaded—glassware.

Looking beyond glassware to other dishes and serving pieces, we can see the potential for lead content. Any vintage metal dishes, or any suspect paint around the home can easily be tested for lead content. If you have any concerns over the material, purchase an inexpensive lead test kit at your local hardware store. Mugs and other dishware that are not microwave safe likely have lead in the ceramic glaze or clay. Another reason for not being microwave safe is metallic decorative glaze. If made in Asia they are typically leaded and hazardous as they can leach lead with heat from the microwave. An additional way to know that something is not microwave safe is if you heat it in the microwave with food or liquid and the dish ends up hotter than the contents. Goods containing lead paint are often very brightly colored as a clue to their heavy metal coating. Domestic made pottery is lead free and more eco-conscious producers exclusively make heavy metal free products.

Another heavy metal with a questionable presence in our home is mercury. Kitchen thermometers with metallic fluid contents should be disposed of at your local hazardous waste disposal event, usually at no cost. The chance for fluids to include mercury is high in the US, whereas in Europe, mercury is banned from production in household thermometers. In contrast, a digital readout thermometer allows for fast reads and you can leave it on the stove without worry of glass or mercury contamination if they should be damaged. A mercury compound is also found in high fructose corn syrup. This heavy metal, even in trace amounts, accumulates in all tissues in our bodies. This metal impairs cognitive function and is a potential cancer causing agent. If your choice of beverage for a treat is a soda, opt for vintage ones made with refined sugar, stevia, or sparkling fruit juice.

Whole fruits and vegetables help the body to flush heavy metals out of the bloodstream and add great flavor to recipes—naturally—from the inside out. Of course, contact your doctor immediately with any concerns. A well-rounded diet means eating healthfully without increasing toxic exposure. For example, not only is mercury toxin found in thermometers for food and in the processing of high fructose corn syrup, but it is also found in certain "wild" or ocean-caught fish. Sustainable and low in mercury, salmon is one of the best fish to eat. Swordfish, mackerel, sardine, and high quality tuna are high in mercury. The key point is that *the longer the fish lives in the ocean, and the higher the fat content, then the higher the mercury it contains.* That is, *the bigger the fish, the higher the mercury content.*

Mercury levels in ocean fish are just one symptom of a global issue resulting from the many practices for fishing which are harmful for the entire food chain. Techniques that dredge the sea floor, longline fishing, and the use of nets are indiscriminate and are devastating for all creatures, including those inadvertently or accidentally harvested. Local fish, farmed shellfish, and wild standard caught fish for consumption are not generally caught by unethical fishing practices. The fish that are exclusively fished by indiscriminate longlines all have higher mercury content. *By avoiding fish with high mercury you automatically avoid many of the long line caught fish.* Even with the introduction of dolphin-safe tuna, the dolphin populations remain in jeopardy if they are part of the "collateral damage" of net fishing. Switching to the consumption of freshwater fish and fish species found at the Environmental Defense Fund's website, <seafood.edf.org/guide/best/healthy> is ideal for the health of our oceans.

Our waterways are also affected by the cookware we use. Nonstick-coated pans purchased before 2015 give off more toxic carcinogens in chemical vapors when heated above medium. Therefore, heat only to medium heat or avoid using them at all. Also, the manufacture of cookware with a nonstick coating increases levels of perfluorinated chemicals (PFCs) in consumers' water supplies near certain production plants. High blood levels of PFCs are linked to high miscarriage rates in pregnant women. Because PFCs are still in broad use in nonstick, wrinkle free, and water resistant applications on fabrics, fast food packaging, and clothing, they should be banned from production. These uses make the probable list of PFC products proliferate shockingly. It is another widespread chemical that's detrimental to humans, wildlife, and the health of our world's waterways and oceans.

Kitchen tools are an often-overlooked category when switching to organic living. Plastic and nylon cooking tools are another obstacle to going green because they melt at relatively low temperatures and thus end up in foods made with them at even moderate temperatures. Bamboo, stainless steel, wooden, or silicon tools are heatproof at higher temperatures and are non-reactive with foods in general. The combination of plastic cooking tools with toxic nonstick pans used to be standard in all households but it's now possible to use readily available non-PFC pans and natural cooking tools.

Making freezer meals ahead in glass containers with leftovers for work, or for the kids to take to school, is a way around using canned foods. Develop a habit to prepare leftovers for the freezer right after a big meal. In no time, there will be a variety of options in the freezer. Among soups, stews, chicken, rice, and pasta the possibilities are endless and taste fresh. Take lunch to work in a two-cup glass container frozen. It keeps your entire lunch bag cold and is the perfect size for a meal. Simply replace the lid with a paper towel (microwave) or foil (conventional oven) to reheat with ease. For oven heating, cover a slightly defrosted container with foil and bake on a sheet pan for approximately 30 minutes at 350 degrees Fahrenheit. Microwaving takes approximately 15–20 minutes on high to cook from a frozen state, stirring occasionally. For much faster reheating, allow it to defrost in the refrigerator overnight and cook on high for three to five minutes. Using glass containers, disposable paper containers, or microwave safe ceramic containers for microwave meals is than heating food in disposable plastic bowls, common in many homes.

If every item that entered the home had a label listing its chemical additives and how they could harm or affect us, we would have greater peace of mind. Being an informed consumer sometimes means reading between the lines, but that is no way to live. There are business practices in every aspect of food production that have a chance for improvement for the health of everyone.

What Else is in Your Food?

Food additives, in small enough amounts, don't need to be reported to the FDA or listed on package labels. That is how and why certain contaminants, chemicals, food dyes, and heavy metals can be hidden from consumers. Chemicals like BHT, also known as TBHQ and BHA, are petroleum-based preservatives in mass produced foods. Its initial purpose was as a preservative in jet fuel and other petroleum products. Avoid products packaged with this chemical and other preservative agents, such as in fast food and beauty products. This is another chemical unsafe for human consumption due to its carcinogenic properties.

Arsenic is another harmful contaminant in food. It is leached from the environment in certain foods more than others. Indeed, this known poison in liquid or concentrated form is a favorite killer in murder mysteries. Some untreated water-cultivated crops such as rice and seaweed are higher in heavy metals due to their innate water filtering nature which helps to clean the water they are grown in, but which means that they retain high levels of the toxins they have removed from their environment. Pesticides and herbicides are also absorbed by these crops. Limiting your rice or seaweed consumption to one to two servings a week lessens your exposure. In cases of eating rice due to gluten intolerance, gluten-free bread and potatoes can substitute. Domestic sources of rice and seaweed in the west are traditionally lower in toxins and metals than foreign brands. For rice specifically, Indian and California grown basmati rice are the lowest in arsenic.

Carrageenan is also a potential carcinogen found in milk and other thickened beverages and foods. It's heavily processed and degraded from seaweed and is known to have carcinogenic properties. It's even found in some organic products and commonly consumed beverages. This emulsifier and thickener can irritate the digestive system and inflame the body. Utilizing the recipes below for milk alternatives, buying local, or switching to organic brands without carrageenan are ways to steer clear of this additive.

Petroleum products are utilized in soymilk production and vinegar, too. Certain brands of common vinegar specifically say they don't process with petroleum, but one way to know for sure that it isn't is if the label declares that it's made with grain or some other crop. For cleaning, using organic vinegar or conventional vinegar—without petroleum—is critical to minimizing exposure to petroleum in the kitchen. For healthier alternative versions of mass produced milk, try recipes like these:

Alternative Milk Recipe

1 Part Nuts (Organic Nuts: Almonds, Cashew, or Hazelnut, or Steamed Rice)
3 Parts Water (4 Parts Water if you're making Rice Milk)

Combine in a blender until smooth. Strain through cheesecloth (if you want a smooth texture). Add vanilla extract or raw sugar, as needed. The solids left over from straining are great in baking or for topping cereals. Keep in the refrigerator.

Soy Milk Recipe

1 Cup Cooked Organic Soybeans
10 Cups water

Combine in a blender, adding sugar or natural sweetener to taste (about three tablespoons). Keep refrigerated. If using dried soybeans use 11 cups of water. Soak the beans overnight, then the next day add everything to a stockpot to boil for about four minutes, or until tender. Once cool, purée in a blender, and strain through cheesecloth. Keep in the refrigerator.

As noted earlier, labeling on packaging is the focus of a growing dispute between big corporations and consumers.

Domestic labels are currently not required to list additives such as food dyes, petroleum products, preservatives, sulfites, flavor enhancers, and perfumes (esters that mimic natural flavors). Since the majority of taste is dictated by the sense of smell, ester perfumes are used as unnatural flavorings in many food items and candies. In small enough percentages, ingredients do not have to be reported. GMO ingredients are also not required to be declared on labels. In Europe, artificial dyes, flavors, and GMOs are banned and must comply with stricter labeling standards. Some of these chemicals cause allergic reactions in sensitive individuals, as is the case for Red 4 (FD&C Red No. 4), a dye made from ground-up tiny red insects called cochineal. Some people are allergic to this form of red 4, and others avoid it because it's not vegan. Switching back to real flavors and colors from benign plant sources, as Europe has, is a direction in which some mainstream companies are heading and others will soon follow.

Imports from countries not known for excess chemical use, as in Europe, have been held to higher labeling standards, so cheeses and other foods from Europe that don't have organic labels can be safely assumed as organic in the US. Their stricter guidelines for labeling and farming of produce and animals make for cleaner, healthier products for the consumer.

In Europe artificial food dyes and flavors are banned, yet the US permits them, even though the common domestic food dyes are derived from petroleum. Like other petroleum products they don't belong in food. Preliminary indications link these less-studied additives to behavioral problems in children and are reason enough to avoid candies, treats, and sodas containing them. Lunch bag staples to take to school are loaded with dyes. Kraft has since removed dyes from its top products due to consumer protest. Making trendy red velvet cake or colorful desserts can be done without any food coloring. You can add chocolate décor, glaze, organic flowers, organic fresh fruit, or use an icing comb for added effect without food dyes.

Always use non-reactive cookware for cooking acidic foods. Aluminum reacts to acids by discoloring your food and giving it a tinny taste. Nobody wants a *green* lemon pie filling. On the other hand, stainless steel and enamel-coated cookware won't interact with any contents while cooking. Aluminum does have its uses. Covering baking dishes with aluminum foil prevents excessive browning and dehydrating of the food while being cooked. Take the extra step, when baking and storing acidic dishes like lasagna and enchiladas, to double layering, first with parchment and following with aluminum foil.

Knowing what's in your food staples is a huge step towards organic living. Making healthful choices to stock a kitchen with maximum nutrition and minimum toxins is relatively simple. Besides, seeing food as the lifeline to good health puts proper food choices into perspective. When we make healthy food we feel good, and so will our families.

It is Medicine

Using specific foods as natural alternatives to modern medicine is an ancient practice. To ease joint pain of any sort, eat a snack size bowl of organic frozen fresh cherries, or fresh if you can find them. As we age, we have more aches and pains, and cherries are a natural anti-inflammatory. They can even curb joint pain caused by medications without having to take more medicine. The positive effects cherries have on bodily pains are documented. Onion and garlic have the same effect on the body but with the downside of strong odors. These are prime examples of ways in which food can be healing for the body. However, consult your doctor beforehand, even for small changes in your diet and especially before contemplating any changes in prescription medications.

Ginger is a cost effective and widely available natural remedy for motion- or seasickness without the side effects, including nausea, of commonly taken over-the-counter dimenhydrinate. For gastric health and nausea, a simple hot ginger tea eases symptoms rapidly and is a remedy for morning sickness in some pregnant women. Just add a small spoonful of raw or locally farmed honey for increased stomach relief and a more pleasing taste. Ginger adds a spicy and slightly sweet dimension to soups and stews as well. It is effective as an anti-inflammatory too, and can be a delicious addition to sweet or savory dishes. In the form of candied ginger or ginger candy, it is easy to carry with you while traveling, at work, or on the go. Ginger snaps or gingerbread cookies are kid friendly. Just store them in the freezer to be on hand for occasional stomach ailments.

If your child or family member bites their tongue or cheek, a quick trip to the sugar bowl not only stops minor blood flow, but also a child's tears. Applying ice to the wound has an effect similar to a spoon full of sugar on the tongue or inside a cheek. If your four-legged family member has a small nick, perhaps from accidental over trimming of nails, dip the wound in a small cup of sugar. However, if the bleeding persists contact the proper provider for care.

Another surprising benefit of food derives from the consumption of probiotics in fermented foods, yogurts, and other soured milk products. *There are new studies that suggest they boost mood and improve emotional and digestive health.* They are great for both humans and their pets because domestic animals benefit as we do from probiotics, fiber, fresh fruits and vegetables. The link between gut health and overall brain health is being emphasized more in modern studies of diets for the entire household. One or two servings a day of probiotics for humans and a small amount a day for your pets, with gradual incorporation to avoid stomach upset, is a great way to maximize nutrition. *When taking antibiotics for infection, take a multiple probiotic strain supplement 4 hours after antibiotics, on an empty stomach, to repopulate good bacteria in the body without counteracting the medical effects of the antibiotic.* This helps prevent recurrence of the original infection by boosting good bacteria while sidestepping any weakening of the immune system due to the antibiotics' killing off good bacteria. Probiotic supplements work well when traveling to boost immune health and prevent any traveler's illnesses. Always keep probiotic supplements in the refrigerator maximum bacteria count. In the next chapter we will discuss the link between good bacteria in the body and the severity of allergies.

A cure-all in Asia is turmeric. Taking a spoonful of turmeric in a smoothie or yogurt will shorten the common cold, cure stomach ailments, reduce inflammation, and improve general health. Adding this mild spice to any dish is a good way to sneak it into your diet. One surprising tip is to buy the higher quality organic spices. Lower-quality (perhaps lower-priced) spices tend to have unusual add-ins and chemicals in them so it's worth finding trusted purveyors online or survey the more expensive organic bottles in the grocery spice aisle. When adding spices in large amounts to recipes, or consuming spices for medicinal purposes, choosing organic spices is investing in your health.

Superfood Tricks

New foods are always being touted as the next superfood. Not all superfoods appeal to everyone, but in this section are some recipes and tricks to incorporate them into your diet. The occasional green smoothie or juice improves health. Many people swear by them. A quick trick is to combine kale or spinach with pomegranate juice to mask any bitterness of the greens. Also add some diced fruit, soymilk or yogurt for sweetness and texture. *When consuming large amounts of leafy greens, your body will crave salty foods*. This is because, with the high amount of potassium you're consuming, your body naturally needs salt to process them together for electrolyte balance. The most natural salt is sea salt and consuming it will help boost your daily mineral intake. Be aware of any food cravings. Keep lightly salted organic dry roasted nuts, baked organic vegetable chips (not necessarily potato chips), and homemade sea salt kale chips around for a healthy alternative to fried chips or crackers. With the consumption of excess of vitamin K from kale and other greens, please eat with restraint as it can interfere with blood thinners for those with high blood pressure or other cardiac issues.

Sea Salt Kale Chips

1 Bunch Organic Kale
1-2 Tablespoons Organic Oil (Canola, Vegetable, or Peanut)
¼-½ Teaspoon Sea Salt

Line two sheet pans with parchment. Remove and discard the stems from the kale and tear the leaves into one-inch pieces. Wash and thoroughly dry in a salad spinner. Toss to combine kale with oil and sea salt. Place in a single layer on the baking sheets. On the center racks, bake at 350 degrees Fahrenheit for approximately 15 minutes until the kale lightly browns on the edges.

Buying seasonal organic fruits and vegetables in abundance at their peak is a great way to save money in colder months. Wash and chop individual fruits or vegetables and place on a parchment lined baking sheet in the freezer. Once frozen, pack into containers in the freezer for inexpensive offseason enjoyment. Frozen tropical fruits are a healthy alternative to sweetened popsicles in the summertime and are equally satisfying.

Coconut Chia Pudding

A simple chia pudding is satisfying and a nutrition packed go-to dessert or breakfast. It is a simple and healthy organic recipe to make for any occasion. This superfood is easily found in the bulk bins of your natural market. Instead of coconut milk you can use any milk or dairy alternative.

⅓ Cup Chia Seeds
1 Can Coconut Milk (16 oz.)
3 Tablespoons Maple Syrup (Or Other Natural Sweetener)
½ Teaspoon Vanilla Extract

¼ Cup Water (If Necessary)

Whisk all ingredients in a bowl. If your canned coconut milk has a large layer of coconut cream on top, add an extra quarter cup of water to adjust its consistency or viscosity. Cover and refrigerate overnight. Top with fruit, cocoa powder, nuts or cinnamon for variety and nutrition. Serves four.

Deconstructed Smoothie Parfait

For dessert, breakfast, or snack this smoothie parfait is a quick and portable recipe. It's a virtually mess-free version of a smoothie and more complex with intact layers of flavor.

¾ Cup Yogurt
2 Tablespoons Fruit Juice
½ Cup Fresh or Frozen Fruit
1 Tablespoon Muesli (or Chopped Nuts)
1 Drop Vanilla Extract

Layer yogurt, fruit, drop of vanilla extract, and orange juice in a bowl or Mason jar. Serves one.

Cooperative markets with membership programs offer occasional coupons in the newspaper or online. Most, if not all, of the products they carry are also fair trade exclusive; that is, paid labor was used. Many large food corporations employ child or slave labor to harvest their staple crops for their products. Avoid those companies. This can be difficult to do in supermarkets, as the majority have links to a product in their line that is made with inhumane business practices. The fair trade stamp assures you that the products conform to animal- and human-friendly guidelines, for peace of mind, and can strengthen the direction of ethical food production and influence other industries, as well. The consumer dictates production. If the demand declines for products of corporations that aren't using humane practices, they'll be forced to reassess and adjust both their standards and their practices.

Grocery shopping for your family is easier than ever as many big box and local stores are supplying organic options to fulfill consumer demand. Ask for more products at your local grocery store, if their supply is limited, and they will adjust. Increasing options for you also helps your community. As more people switch to organic due to chemical concerns, more families will benefit. We can all do our part to encourage organic eating as it also helps local farmers. Local farms, just like the farmers markets, supply organic produce to many grocery stores. Unifying the connection between farms and homes allows for nutrient-rich products to reach growing families, and ensures the freshest products for the long haul.

Reaping the rewards of clean eating allows for more energy to be put towards even more meaningful aspects of life. Taking care of family and the home are some of them. In the next chapters will be an array of recipes for alternatives to harsh chemicals in the house. Not adding dangerous chemicals, toxins, or carcinogens to the world's water cycle is beneficial to living, both for the future and the now. Knowing how we are all interconnected by how we live means we can take that extra step to keep the Earth as green as possible.

Family

"If you want to change the world, start with the next person who comes to you in need."

— B. D. Schiers

$\mathcal{M}$aking healthful purchases for your family is a challenge. Be informed and wary of products grown and made overseas in some areas of the world, including clothing and food for our pets and us. Many chemicals banned in the States and Europe are produced freely in Asia. Imported clothing, kitchen items, and food don't have the same standards as locally produced goods, resulting in higher exposure to chemicals and heavy metals. A preference for "Made in America" is a double-edged sword with risks of exposure to heavy chemicals on clothing and in products around your home. With a bit of extra time, and perhaps an extra shopping list, one change at a time leads towards a more organic life beginning with acknowledging the health benefits of natural living. You owe it to yourself in this short lifetime to take care of yourself, certainly, but also your family and household. Start small, whether it be with a single cleaning product or a pantry staple, and soon enough your house will be purified.

Any time spent outdoors is great for you and your family's overall health. Rolling up the sleeves to get your vitamin D for the day is a great way to increase mood and to boost bone health. The combination of sun and fresh air is ideal to re-center oneself and disconnect from stressors. Sunshine is also important for the eyes of a growing fetus, because they are among the last organs to fully develop before birth. Thus there might be more to the *babymoon* than just getting away before a baby's expected arrival. It may help create a deeper connection between the expectant parents, encouraging baby's healthier growth and development while growing up.

Our skin also heals us. The sweat produced from an intense workout or sauna helps to heal skin surfaces. It's nature's topical ointment, when long before modern medicine we had to forage to survive and potentially heal ourselves from the outside in. The incalculable benefits from a good sweat session can push body cleansing to a new level and is worthy of research.

Simplified

Inquiring about what is applied to our skin is made simple with the many online websites that rate the organic nature of an array of commercially produced beauty products. Their databases are vast, but not complete, so it's beneficial to understand the basics of beauty supplies and the chemicals in them. The government is decades behind with household chemical testing for human use, so, when in doubt, err on the side of caution. Utilizing the household care recipes throughout this book helps reduce the use of chemicals that can harm. One word of warning is the FDA does not regulate organic or natural cosmetics such as facial makeup, making the "organic" and "natural" labels meaningless on non-food products, though they aren't necessarily meant to be misleading. It's up to us as educated consumers to research and purchase the brands with the cleanest products.

Parabens, derived from petroleum, are also something people worry about, but luckily there are alternatives. Like all petroleum products, parabens have the potential to have negative effects on the endocrine system, yet they are found in cosmetics and skin care products. They're added to standard makeup and lotions for their ability to act as a moisture barrier for keeping the skin from dehydrating. Some naturally occurring ingredients like beeswax and natural oils have the same effect. Great organic product lines that are amazing for your skin are readily found at spas and natural markets. I find that alternative organic lotions work better than mass-market lotions. For an even skin tone and the reduction of wrinkles, look for lotions with hyaluronic acid, also called hyaluronan, naturally occurring in fruits and vegetables. The top skincare lines incorporate wild versions in their lotions and cleansers.

More troubling for skincare are the heavy metals in mass produced makeup. Your local health food store will have options for natural makeup that are petroleum and heavy metal free. Some people find organic makeup to be dehydrating, as they are all natural, so they don't apply as easily. To allow for a smoother finish, you can add a drop of organic argan oil to your makeup, or apply the oil directly to the skin as a moisturizer before applying makeup. Test on a small spot on your face to make sure your skin isn't sensitive to this treatment. Another option for smoothing out natural makeup is adding a daily moisturizer to your foundation to achieve the same ease.

Other salon chemicals that are a focus of concern include hair dyes and other colorants, among the several hair altering products commonly available. More salons are popping up that take an organic approach. Consumers realize the dangers of harmful chemicals floating around the typical salon, and want a safer environment for their beauty needs. Hair dyes contain chemicals with volatile organic compounds (VOCs) and other carcinogens. Though they are caustic they are widespread in salons. With an increasing demand for natural alternatives for conventional beauty treatments, there are more options than ever for salons that are up to organic standards.

One worrisome chemical derived from petroleum is sodium lauryl sulfate (SLS). It pollutes our waters and is a fungicide and insecticide. As we will discuss more about fungicides later in the book, it is alarming the FDA allows this chemical in mass production. This foaming agent is found often in toothpaste and in shampoo. Several years ago there were natural toothpaste options with calcium sodium phosphosilicate (CSP) on the market. CSP is a bio glass that repairs and restores enamel and prevents tartar buildup and sensitivity. It's basically the safest and therefore the best thing for oral health on the market. Since the incorporation of CSP into toothpastes, a big US corporation has pulled all products containing CSP from the shelves after having bought the patent. The products pulled had CSP, were fluoride-free and SLS-free (sodium lauryl sulfate, mentioned earlier). Several companies had been making this natural version of toothpaste but all brands have now stopped production. It had superior components compared to other natural products, which are known for their highly abrasive qualities. The next best option is buying sensitivity toothpaste from Europe or Canada. They have the bio glass in them, but they do contain fluoride and SLS. If tooth sensitivity isn't a problem for you, then carefully brushing with a natural toothpaste is the best alternative.

To avoid SLS in hair products, natural markets have stocked an array of natural shampoo and conditioner options in the bulk bins and in their beauty aisle. Below is a natural recipe for convenience.

Shampoo

1 Cup Water
1 Cup Liquid Castile Soap (made from vegetable fats)

Shake to combine in a stoppered bottle. Apply to scalp and massage in. Condition with store bought natural conditioner or with a dime size amount of argan oil.
Note: Argan Oil can also be used as a heat protectant before styling on wet or dry hair in the same amount.

Makeup Remover

Jojoba Oil, Olive Oil, or Vegetable Oil
Cotton Cosmetic Pads

Apply oil to a cotton pad and gently blot away makeup. Follow with your favorite soap or cleanser and with your favorite moisturizer.

Note: In my family, the line of women before me all have beautiful skin. They always apply moisturizer or sunscreen to their hands and face in the morning and at night. This simple routine along with proper makeup removal encourages a youthful appearance with ease.

One of the most problematic chemicals in the powder room of many homes is found in antibacterial soaps, mass market toothpastes, hand sanitizers, and detergents: triclosan (triclocarban). Years after initial production of triclosan soap for homes across the world, it was discovered in the late 1970s to impact fertility negatively. The FDA only recently banned this substance and other antibacterials in soaps, but is still allowed in other products. This controversial soap ingredient is now known to cause hormone imbalances. Since triclosan has antifungal properties, this isn't surprising. In the final chapter we will discuss more about fungi in the home and how we're more related to fungi than we are to plants. Antifungal ingredients in foods and in cleansers are red flags for consumers. They should be classified as too toxic to be in the home. Your skin is the biggest organ in the body; it's important not to expose yourself to triclosan. It can also start puberty early and increase infertility risk. This should be eliminated from production and use. Until then, check the labels on your toiletries and opt for some alternatives like Castile soap and moisturizing milk soaps from local or natural purveyors. Hand washing with regular soap is as effective as antibacterial soap when applied the same way. Triclosan and alcohol based hand sanitizers contribute to the evolution of superbugs, microbes resistant to traditional cleansing methods, by permitting only the most robust microbes to survive and to reproduce. Washing our hands with natural soap is a way not to contribute to this microscopic dilemma.

Surprisingly, the vast majority of standard soap bars for the body and face are made with tallow, a waxy byproduct of the meat industry, making the bar soaps neither vegan nor growth hormone or antibiotic free. Who would have thought there could be antibiotics and growth hormones in your bar soaps? Vegetable oil based soaps instead of tallow soaps are easily available online and in specialty stores. They make great gifts and can be an opportunity for sharing these lesser-known facts about the soap industry.

A not-so-surprising chemical that also interferes with necessary bodily functions is found in antiperspirants. The aluminum compounds found in them prevent sweat glands from excreting elements from the body around the underarm. Antiperspirants have been linked to breast cancer in women due to their prevention of lymph nodes from flushing with normal sweating. Anything the body would normally excrete though the lymphatic system stays within the closed internal system. Natural deodorants don't block any flow of sweat while effectively masking odors, and are therefore an ideal alternative.

More Than Skin Deep

Chemicals such as preservatives, dyes, and PFCs with carcinogenic properties are used in the production of standard clothing. Fabrics treated for wrinkle resistance and stain resistance contain carcinogenic chemicals, PFCs, that can't be washed away. Cotton is currently a GMO and is one of the most heavily sprayed crops. The toxic chemicals sprayed on the fields are even more harmful than those on corn and soy. Historically, cotton had been sprayed with lead and arsenic based insecticide which remains in the soil for years after initial application. Organic cotton clothing and feminine products may be found online and in specialty shops. If it's not financially possible to buy organic clothing make sure you wash all clothing and cloth items well, especially before first use. Knowing what you're really buying is more important than the ease of care for a piece of clothing by not having to iron. Fabrics of cotton, silk, cashmere, and other natural fibers all allow for maximum skin breathing. Our skin is our largest organ and, because its surface is semipermeable, our pores absorb chemicals from clothing and our environment, especially in warm weather.

One such contaminant is nicotine. Infants, children, and adults absorb nicotine from their environment and from particles on skin. Numerous studies have shown that any use of nicotine by relatives ends up in children's bloodstreams. These same children weren't exposed to second hand smoke or direct use; they only received contact from microscopic transfer (third hand smoke). This carcinogenic source is now known to be harmful in microscopic forms on surfaces long after the actual smoke was suspended in the air space. This toxic dust is one lesser-known example of carcinogens in our environment. The increasing awareness of the devastating and damaging effects of smoking has reduced rates of harm on behavior and health.

The presence of these virtually unknown chemicals and compounds, at least to large portions of our citizenry, exemplifies the need for a higher stance from the large companies and beyond. Their moral responsibility should be to eliminate production of harsh or unethical chemicals in place of Earth-friendly alternatives. If we stop buying products containing such harmful ingredients, we can change the direction of chemical use in these mass-produced everyday items.

Hypoallergenic Tricks

Beneficial bacteria can keep the immune system from having the hyper alert functions that are known as allergies. *The more we use super chemicals, the higher the frequency of allergies,* especially in children. Letting kids play in the dirt, and being exposed to more bacteria, decreases their risk in later life for developing autoimmune disorders. It can be inferred that super cleaner use, over a prolonged period of time, increases the risk for autoimmune disorders. Allow your body's beneficial bacteria to repopulate your digestive system and skin by eliminating super cleaners and harsh chemicals around the home. Add good bacteria in your gut by consuming the probiotic rich foods and supplements discussed in the previous chapter. Good bacteria aid digestion and general health of the body. Good bacteria in the mouth are also shown to help break foods down before they even reach the stomach. These beneficial bacteria also can displace many harmful bacteria that have the potential to settle in the blood stream and the heart. Good oral health is another building block for optimal general health. *Natural and non-antibacterial toothpastes encourage good bacteria to flourish and discourage bad bacteria from settling in the gum line.* Beneficial bacteria's impact on overall health exemplifies the need for eliminating super cleaners from the home.

Using heat as a way to eliminate dust mite allergens is a natural method of allergy reduction. Washing and drying your bedding on high heat greatly reduces dust mites. Hypoallergenic linens are an available online option. They fully encapsulate mattresses and pillows and are mite-proof barriers.

For other allergies like hay fever, brush your teeth twice a day with a sensitivity toothpaste that contains *potassium nitrate,* which even in such minute amounts works well for most people as an antihistamine. Another dental care note: for those with rounded teeth, woven floss works the best to maximize floss coverage around all curves of the teeth between the gum line. A dentist once told me not to use plastic film-floss as it simply "glides around plaque and buildup." Even though dental practices might give away samples of it for free, there's a reason they don't use the product on you during your visit. Woven floss or standard floss is the best option. Always brush with an electric toothbrush, at any price point, to gain a mechanical advantage for tooth care. And of course, gently brush your tongue, gums, and cheeks.

Later in the book we will discuss the benefits of natural cleaning over conventional chemicals' link to allergies and other immune system issues. The recipes will focus on the main chemicals we traditionally use around the home.

Connection with your Pets

Pets will appreciate chemical-free living. For any animals with sensitive skin, you may notice a reduction in scratching after ceasing the use of a chemical-laced solution for skincare, bathing, or pest control. That's assuming a veterinarian deemed the pet healthy prior to this. Keeping your pets happy with fresh water and the occasional treat is simple. Before adding anything new to your pet's diet always ask your veterinarian. But in general dogs love the following vitamin boosting treats: baby carrots, green beans, and broccoli. The longest living cats and dogs ate broccoli daily, and if you can get your pets to enjoy it, great! Initially, cut or break all treats into small pieces to ensure that your pets respond well to training. Besides, it's a wonderful way to bond and build a mutually respectful relationship with your pet.

In building this mutual respect, it's imperative to establish boundaries and proper manners. Pets thrive off boundaries and if they do something you don't like there's an unorthodox trick. For both dogs and cats snap your fingers at the first sign of a behavior you want to stop. It might be their posture, like they're going to jump on the kitchen table or the desk full of papers. Instead of saying "no" it tells them exactly what you don't like. The sharp and slightly loud noise with a quick command following, like "off," works without conditioning a response from your voice. Quickly add praise once they complete the desired behavior. Eventually you can say the command and only supplement with the snap if they're not responding. When we first adopted our older cat from the shelter I didn't want him to associate "no" from my voice when scolding him. For over five years we've used this snapping technique and he understands exactly the boundaries we set for him. Originally, we had a spray bottle with water to "teach him" where he could and couldn't go, but it felt too harsh. He would run away in fear. I knew there had to be a better option. I started snapping my fingers instead and I got a response of a sassy meow. I'd rather have a cat talk back to me than run away in fear. I soon tested it on the family's elderly dog and she had a better reaction too as she was desensitized to the word "no" from being spoiled by her human parents for too long. Mutual respect between you and your pet deepens your connection and ensures the possibility of future training.

One of the fastest ways to train your pet is to find their favorite foods. This is a fun game the kids can help with. It shows them the discipline and portion control responsibilities of taking care of another being and teaches empathy. Make sure to educate the family about foods pets can't have. For dogs and cats prohibited foods include cherries, avocado, grapes, garlic, onion, coffee, tea, candy, xylitol, and chocolate products. These should be avoided as well: fats, dairy, spices, and pork. Dogs can have some dairy, but always introduce it in small amounts to test for intolerance. With dogs, take a more alpha dog approach and only allow them to try some after the meal is over and put away. Some cats are very food driven and also need these same boundaries. Feeding high quality food ensures healthy living for our fur babies, both cats and dogs. With the help of the veterinarian, find high quality wet and dry foods that your pet enjoys. Adding canned pumpkin, other vegetable purées, or diced vegetable boosts the nutrients for both species. Gradually introducing one new food at a time is easier on their stomachs and for finicky eaters. Once their favorite foods are established, they will try their hardest to learn how they might continue to reap the rewards of their good behavior.

Channeling any excess energy your pet may have is beneficial to their health. For pets that were once strays, the tactics they once had to utilize to find a meal in the wild needs a proper outlet or they'll find new games to play. Letting them outside on leashed walks works well with both cats and dogs. This lessens any neuroticism from being indoors and creates a more mentally balanced cat or dog. For cats, even 10 minutes leashed on the back patio is sufficient to fulfill this outdoor need. Leashed time outside is especially necessary for cat breeds not suited for outdoor life as they are ill equipped to defend themselves. They learn to trust you, to follow your lead, and they get to explore with more than just their eyes. A full mix of sensory stimuli allows your pet to flourish and be calmer when indoors.

A cat happy outside and inside the home is easy to achieve by making sure they have access to good quality litter. The litter your cat walks through multiple times daily is ideally made with natural materials. Those made with cracked wheat are naturally odor reducing and clump well. Wheat litters are free of clay, baking soda, and fragrance, which are all important considerations for cat litter. The compounds in standard litter are hard on cat's kidneys and switching to natural is easy for cats. Gradually incorporating new litter allows them to acclimate.

Another approach to pet bonding is meditation. Pet ownership and meditation bring youth back to your life, help reduce blood pressure, and together bring peace to you and your pet. Pets are sensitive and enjoy the calm when in deep meditation. It might take practice but soon they too will sit in silence and enjoy this quiet bonding time. Depending on the energy level of the pet, sitting in a chair, on the floor, on a pillow, or outside in the sun are some great options. Starting at a few minutes a day, fitting in this "me time" is energizing and rejuvenating to settle the chaos of the mind.

Knowing what we know about going green is relatively simple for bringing peace to the home. There are many opportunities for making new choices for you and your family, but if they don't feel comfortable for you, it's okay. There are always new options hitting the market or different choices you can make. Only you know what's best for your family's needs. Treating every daily event as an opportunity to find peace is a skill we can all try to master. In the next chapter, there are tips to eating anything you want with peace of mind.

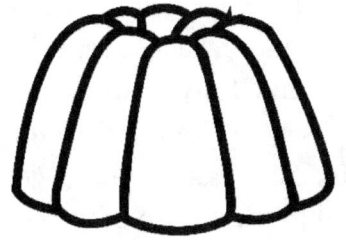

Nutrition Tips

"The first wealth is health."

—Ralph Waldo Emerson

$\mathcal{M}$y father and I met with a dietitian to attempt to reverse his diagnosis of pre-diabetes at age 60. He followed the guidelines below and lost 40 pounds and is now healthier than ever and, more important, diabetes free. It was difficult for him, at first, to take a step back and look at his eating habits because he grew up in a time when it wasn't known how portion control and good fats were important considerations in daily meals. He began counting calories, and weighing his food, so he could see exactly what he was eating. He consciously started making decisions about the meals he was preparing. Between exercising five days a week and this lifestyle switch, he has since been able to maintain for the past year. He is still finding a balance so he doesn't have to count calories anymore. Over the past two years he learned not to beat himself up over eating a bad meal, not count calories all the time, that good fat isn't bad for you, how to throw food away when full, not to obsess about the little things, and to enjoy his new found health. This plan also helps to avoid blood sugar crashes as it is designed for maximum satiety and efficiency. These tips aren't just for weight loss and are great to adapt into your diet for healthy filling options. As always, before attempting major changes in your diet contact your healthcare professional to ensure safety for your specific health needs.

These are foods and fats that are good for you and are simple to add to your diet:

Nuts
Nut butters
Avocado
Coconut oil
Legumes
Beans
Whole wheat sprouted bread.
2% or low fat cheeses
Whole eggs
Low fat Greek yogurt

High fiber cereal

Sugar alternatives for those with pre diabetes or diabetes: xylitol and stevia are very sweet, so use these sparingly in recipes. If the recipe calls for one cup of sugar use one teaspoon of stevia or a ratio of 48:1. With sugar to xylitol the ratio is more like 1.5:1. Xylitol can have a chemical taste if used in excess so make sure you don't over sweeten it, as it can go up to an even ratio.

The tricks in this chapter are simple and very customizable. We will further discuss the benefits and disadvantages of certain food choices in the next chapter.

Can I Still Eat My Favorite Foods?

Stress hormones from beating yourself up for eating junk food only add to the waistline, perpetuating a vicious cycle. Understanding how to eat your favorite foods in a well-rounded way takes any guilt and stress out of eating fast food. Substitutions or changes to American favorites like bread, burgers, and bacon are easy to apply to all cheat foods.

Bacon is low in protein but high in salt and fat. It's recommended to have two slices a month or one slice once or every other week. One trick to avoid temptation and overeating is the fry and freeze method. Fry the entire pack of bacon in whole or cut up bacon pieces, until crisp. Drain on a paper towel, let cool, and freeze in a glass container. When you need one piece, place a piece of bacon in a frying pan on medium low heat. Allow slow defrosting then frying to a crisp, flipping once. This makes the bacon fry faster and is almost mess free, especially if the same (nonstick) pan is used to fry eggs afterwards.

Common breads, bananas, and corn have a high glycemic index and can cause blood sugar spikes just like cake or candy can. They are both pure sugar when processed by the body. Have a half of a banana or a serving of popcorn, on rare occasions. Bread with whole wheat and sprouted seeds maximizes nutrients and slows down digestion.

Switching to grass fed beef, bison or venison hamburgers is a good alternative to greasy take out. Grass fed milk products, including butter, grass fed beef, and other grass fed animal products have omega three fatty acids from the animals' green diet. This ensures maximum nutritional benefit and boosts flavor. Standard corn feed doesn't provide the same nutrition. The flavor in grass fed products is also superior but is best to try it yourself. For example, European or Irish butter especially is packed with flavor. Have a small serving of sweet potato fries to bump up the fiber and vitamin content over regular potato fries.

For meals out at friends' homes and it's not possible to change the menu, serve yourself less so you eat less. In doing so, you save room for a small piece of dessert. These methods for eating "cheat" foods in a healthier way can easily be adapted to any favorite food.

The menu ideas teach portion control in a very manageable way and limit the need for calorie counting. Have a snack an hour or two before bed to prevent blood sugar crashes in the morning. Another trick is to eat a snack 30 minutes before bed in colder months. Your body's digestion will keep you warm through the night. This menu allows easy to make substitutions based on dietary restrictions or preferences. The food staples can be combined and replaced easily for variety. Snacking between meals and not skipping meals keeps the metabolism running, which burns more calories than skipping meals. Below are some meal and snack options for an average 1550-calorie day, give or take 50 calories.

Healthy Snacks

Option 1: One to two tablespoons of peanut butter (or other nut butter) on whole-wheat toast.

Option 2: A serving of cheese and crackers (with about 3g of fiber per serving) and low fat cheese.

Option 3: A piece of fruit.

Option 4: A handful of dry roasted nuts.

Option 5: A serving of low-fat Greek yogurt with berries.

Flexible Meal Ideas

Breakfast

Option 1: 1-2 whole eggs poached with one or two slices of whole grain bread with a piece of low fat sausage.

Option 2: Cereal boosted with 10 g of protein with milk to cover.

Lunch or Dinner

Option 1: Sandwich with lunchmeat and low-fat cheese on whole-wheat bread.

Option 2: Chef's salad with any combination of spinach, lettuce, beans, garbanzo beans, edamame, leftover chicken, sprouts, or cucumber.

Option 3: A bowl of hearty bean soup perhaps enhanced with mirepoix (diced celery, onion, and carrot).

Option 4: A choice from among a whole skinless chicken breast, two chicken thighs, salmon, fish, beef, or pork loin with one cup of brown rice, quinoa or whole-wheat pasta. Sweet potatoes, peas, and other fresh or cooked vegetables should take up two-thirds of the plate for any meal.

Easy Tricks for Healthy Eating

A high-quality lean protein source is eggs. They are high in vitamins, especially in vitamin D and vitamin B-12. There is a stigma around dietary cholesterol yet there is no correlation between dietary cholesterol in eggs and "bad" cholesterol in our bodies. Typically high levels of bad cholesterol are linked to stress, genetics, eating "bad" fats, fried food, and so on. Bad fats come from sources like meat, trans fats from cooking with low smoke point oils, and fat in corn fed dairy products. (In the next section we'll discuss cooking methods without the use of trans fats.)

As an aid to digestion, a glass of low fat or fat free milk with your meal helps to prevent the absorption of some of the bad fats entering the intestines. Having just over two servings of dairy a day meets most calcium requirements for all age groups. Leafy greens, like in the recipe for kale chips in the "Superfood Tricks" section, are also a vegan source of calcium. However, be aware of the recommended daily values of calcium for your gender and age range when calculating your daily calcium allowance, since overconsumption could be a problem, and always consult your doctor before adding new supplements to your daily regimen. One side effect of this surprising fat reducing technique is the prevention of heartburn from spicy or greasy foods.

As more people are avoiding gluten due to dietary restrictions, the array of options is endless due to the easily accessible alternatives to wheat flour. Even most local bakeries have gluten free options that expand beyond bread into sweets and pastries. One healthy option is whole-wheat sourdough bread, which naturally contains less gluten than traditional breads. The yeast in slow fermentation digests the wheat into smaller components and breaks down most of the gluten. Slow risen sourdough has the least amount of gluten because of the extra time allowed for the yeast enzymes to work. Another alternative is spelt flour, the king of alternatives to wheat flour, giving bread a pleasing slightly sweet taste from the grain itself.

To burn extra calories by boosting your metabolic rate is as simple as adding spicy mustard to your sandwich, to marinades, salad dressing, or sauce. Mustard can bump your metabolism and enable you to burn calories faster.

Calorie-cutting tricks are surprisingly easy to pick and choose. These are simple tools in the toolbox for changing the mindset when it comes to meal preparation. For instance, serve foods using smaller plates and eating utensils for better portion control and to enhance slower, mindful eating. Drink plenty of water before, during, and after a meal to aid digestion and to feel full faster. A low-calorie soup before a meal also helps to reduce consumption during the meal.

Surprising Ways to Increase Flavor in Any Recipe

Creating flavor with cooking techniques and changing preparation methods makes even the simplest recipes stand out. See the recipe for roasted tomatoes below as a basic example of building flavor. After roasting, the tomatoes are ready to be used for roasted tomato soup, pasta sauce, or as a side dish on its own. Before adding liquids for a soup or sauce, include a diced tomato, caramelized low and slow, to the mirepoix to enhance the hearty flavor of any vegetarian dish. Another enhancement is *replacing simple carbohydrates like pasta or cornbread with the sweetness and texture of spaghetti squash or sweet potato,* especially when steamed or baked because they pair well with any sauce or chili. They are all high in fiber and low in calories, yet are quite gratifying and satisfying to eat.

Roasted Tomatoes

1 Pound Organic Quartered Roma Tomatoes
½ Teaspoon Organic Oregano, Fresh or Dried
Organic Vegetable Oil
Salt and pepper

Place tomatoes on a sheet pan in a single layer. Lightly drizzle oil and sprinkle on seasonings. Bake at 375 degrees Fahrenheit for 15–20 minutes, or until lightly brown.

Note: Inexpensive half size sheet pans, perfect for any conventional home oven or toaster oven, are available at restaurant supply stores and shops that cater to businesses, and are indispensable for entertaining and streamlined cookie baking.

With the wide variety of cooking shows and videos out there, it's important to examine their directions for healthier living because some advice is not based on scientific or tested experience. For instance, many recipes suggest you brown food on high heat in olive oil. However, this is one oil that shouldn't be cooked with, as its smoke point is so low that the oil will turn into trans fats very quickly, and ingestion of trans fats is linked to depression, among other effects. Stay physically and mentally healthy by using peanut oil, coconut, or other vegetable oils for the high smoke point, and brown food on medium heat instead. To boost flavor add tomato paste, caramelized onion, mirepoix, or vegetable stock. Olive oil is best as a finishing oil, great in salad dressings or topping whole-wheat pasta after cooking. Coconut oil is packed with healthy fats and can be a substitute for butter in baking recipes. Vegetable oil can also be substituted in equal parts for butter. If the oil will produce trans fats when used for cooking, remember that *if the cooking fat changes flavor when heated, it will produce trans fats at lower temperatures.* For example, butter will burn if left on heat for too long, and olive oil loses its signature taste when heated.

There are many other foods to avoid. They cause sugar highs and lows for even the average healthy person. Granola, sweet marinades on meats, fruit juices, white bread, sweetened yogurt, too much milk, and sugary creamy dressings (French, thousand island, or honey mustard), can all cause food cravings after the blood sugar spikes and dips. Thinking twice about the ingredients in the foods we eat and how the body processes them make food choices that much easier.

The switch to healthy choices is based on high protein, the good fats, fiber, nutrients, and satiety. Incorporating any or all of these examples of good food choices will increase energy, decrease blood sugar spikes, and increase overall vitality. There are also other perks, such as improved good cholesterol and reduced bad cholesterol. The more rainbow colors of vegetables and fruits in your diet, the better you will feel while sustaining a healthy body. Besides, locally procured fresh produce and groceries tend to be more flavorful as well as being more nutritious for their freshness. Creating great tasting food from great tasting ingredients is simple. You can substitute according to your tastes and your health needs. It's a highly adaptable menu.

This doesn't mean that you can't eat convenience foods. It's about making better decisions and not creating more stress in your life. As long as there is protein in any cheat meal or snack, know that it is providing nutrition. Many times I've seen friends or family eat bad tasting food because "it's good for you" (and avoiding good tasting food because "it's bad for you"), but the goal is to make *good* tasting food also good for you. The bread aisle at the local grocery store already might have whole wheat, high fiber, and low sugar options. If your grocery store doesn't have these stocked regularly, ask customer service because they take customer requests for items on shelves seriously to bring back customers. The better their inventory matches their customers' needs, the better their business does. Take any stress out of changes by seeing a natural organic regimen not as a diet but as a lifestyle. There aren't any radical restrictive elements like a diet would have, yet it embraces so many alternatives and concessions that there is no reason to feel or be deprived.

Combining many food choice changes, applying subtle twists, and adding good fats and fiber can increase your well-being while adding interesting variety to your weekly menu. When you take care of yourself, your vitality increases and so will your family's. With the example you set for healthy eating and proper self-care, your family will soon see the great progress you're making and want to join you. Discussions about healthy food choices can begin, or continue, so your family will step on and follow a path to good health. It isn't easy to reverse pre-diabetes, especially at age 60 or later, but use it as inspiration and motivation for your own track towards healing yourself from the inside out.

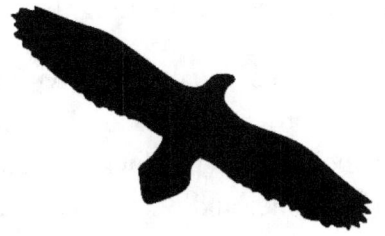

Self-Care

Do not seek to follow in the footsteps of the wise. Seek what they sought.

—Matsuo Basho

*I*nfluence others by living in a peaceful state. Those around you will want to try the same life changes as they see it affecting you in a positive way. You don't have to push them; instead, guide them into healthy life practices to manage stress, increase satisfaction with life, and achieve overall peace. Begin by being kind to yourself and taking care of yourself. Make yourself a priority and your family will mimic your self-reliance and care. Taking a little extra time for self-care yields a feeling of satisfaction and readiness for anything the day brings.

Meditation increases a sense of peace with self, life, and the future, and many work environments are introducing meditation groups, and seeing increases in productivity and creativity. Everyone deserves the inner and outer peace that can be attained with daily practice. Non-denominational meditation like yoga, Pilates, stretching, breathing and relaxation exercises are all viable ways to peace. Limiting added pressures on yourself by reducing the list of "must do" things can reduce stress and increase happiness with your current state.

If you don't feel like you have enough time for a full meditation or relaxation session, a couple of minutes per day would be a good start. Learning to become entranced with silence will result in the natural byproducts of tranquility and contentment—peace and happiness. Meditation can also foster a youthful appearance and acts as a reset button for your tumultuous emotions. Those who meditate rave about its benefits and want you to feel as they do.

Another part of organic living is to live and be the best version of yourself. People go through many breakthroughs in their life where they try to find deeper meaning to their existence. It's already been stated many times but it also means living authentically—discovering then living your life purpose. Use your imagination. What would you do if you had all the time and money in the world? The answer can help you uncover your true purpose. The lucky ones are already doing what they love in a form of hobby, work, or volunteering. Everyone strives to be passionate about what they do, and figuring out how to help other people while enjoying your passion, perhaps in providing a useful product, can lead to a life of fulfillment. With the many resources on the internet and social media, you can sell products or teach classes in your field of expertise. Writing about your passion is also a form of relaxation. Keep a daily journal during downtime. Creative outlets can be therapeutic by redirecting wasteful energies for stress management towards calm management. Creative writing can help revitalize your outlook on life and supply a fresh new perspective.

Always think of yourself first. At first, this seems selfish but doing so will expose your global view. The life you lead has a path that is so broad that the people most important to you can walk with you, all abreast. The important others will be eating the most wholesome foods available while enjoying the health that comes from chemical-free food, heavy-metal and petroleum-free products. Though the long-term effects are impossible to qualify or to quantify, generations after us will have the resources to live in a world that embodies ideals for the betterment of society and the environment. For now, teaching these important life lessons is a public health issue due to our mass consumption of heavily processed foods. Being the healthiest you can be could influence everyone in all communities in a global ripple effect. Your friends, family and others will see the foods you choose to buy, the products chosen for use in your home, and will consider new alternatives. Healthier living is possible for everyone. By leading the way for changes in our eco-consciousness we can help the world.

Around the Home

"There is nothing like staying at home for real comfort."

—Jane Austen

*L*iving for your health now, and for generations to come, includes using products in the home that are good for you and for the environment. If something doesn't appeal to you there are always other options. This isn't meant to be a "must do everything this way or that way," but as a means to expand your options to help keep your home chemical free, yet still clean.

The natural recipes in this chapter are great for people with allergies or chemical sensitivity, as they don't include harsh chemicals or fragrances. Pets and children are especially sensitive to additives and chemicals in fabric softeners, soaps, and detergents. The recipes that follow are safe recipes for families, including pets. Small tasks can add up into one beautifully running organic household. Look at the labels of the cleaners, soaps, and detergents in the home. If there are unnatural fragrances, dyes, or harsh chemicals not meant for skin contact, it's time for them to go. You might see allergies in adults, pets, and children increase with harsh cleaner use. All the ingredients for the family-safe household products below are conveniently found at your local grocery store. This book isn't meant to dismiss any organic products out there, as they are safe, but you will save time and money by making your own cleaning products.

Keep a screen shot photo on your phone or tablet of the tips and recipes you find helpful. Flag the photo as a favorite in your camera roll for on-the-go reference. Make changes easy and accessible with the added benefit of cutting back on paper use by using phone apps. Incorporating the changes is easier to implement when information is nearby. When in doubt keep an extra list handy in your purse or pocket.

Sunshine is nature's disinfectant. It shines away bacteria and viruses effectively and simply with both natural heat and ultra-violet rays. Air drying dishes, clothes, and towels is a great energy saver and supplementally humidifies a home in drier climates, but in excess it contributes to mold and mildew

60

growth in damper climates. In the prevention of toxic mold and its airborne spores in a closed environment such as a well-insulated home, it's important for you and your family to assess whether you need a dehumidifier. Running your bathroom fan for 20-30 minutes during and after showering, or cleaning, will also help to remove the moisture that spores thrive in. Check your baseboards and around windows for signs of mold and, if necessary, clean it with the following mixture:

Natural Mold Cleaner

12 Drops Tea Tree Oil
2 Tablespoons Liquid Castile Soap
1 Cup Warm Water
2-Cup Disposable Container
Paper Towels or Cloth Rags
1 Plastic Bag for Disposal of Waste Paper

Send all pets and family out of the room while cleaning and wear a mask and gloves to prevent contact with spores. Combine and apply the first three ingredients to affected areas with a paper towel or a cloth rag and apply to all moldy surfaces gently until clean. Discard the towel into a waste bag and treat the next area with a new towel. Once all surfaces are treated, place all contaminated items in the bag and tie up to throw away. Allow to dry completely with windows open for ventilation.

Using natural versions of mold and mildew cleaner is a way to avoid the heavily toxic chemicals that are commonly found in shower and bathtub cleaners. Since mildew and mold are forms of fungus, these chemical-laden cleaners are especially harmful to our families. As stated in the second chapter, *we are, after all, more closely related to fungi than we are to plants.*

Standard shower cleaners are essentially killing our lungs and any skin cells the chemical comes in contact with. Toxic fungicides say specifically not to get on skin or to breathe it in, but spraying it in the home might be impossible. To avoid using chemicals on your shower, treat new showers with a clear film liner that prevents hard water and mildew stains. Consult your contractor about applying this film before ordering any new glass shower panels. Also, regularly using microfiber cloths and squeegees after showering prevents glass and tile staining.

To clean mold, dust, or allergens from the air, utilize the box fan and home air filter technique. Bungee cord a new home central air filter to the back of a box fan and run on high. These inexpensive particulate air filters are used in hospitals and care settings. They are ozone free and energy efficient. Ionizing air purifiers and most air conditioning units add ozone to the lower atmosphere, and contribute to global warming. There are ecofriendly brands of air conditioners and purifiers that are noted not to ionize the air, which is a smarter purchase for the environment. Ozone causes adverse reactions, especially for those with respiratory impairments. There are more expensive, but convenient, circular particulate filters online that cover a specific square footage. These are optimal for larger spaces as they circulate the air with greater force. These filters keep the air pure in any environment. Utilizing fresh air and particulate filters is another path to peace of mind in the home.

Fresh air is often contaminated by other products we bring inside the home. Leather polish, PVC shower curtains, and nail polish are common items in the home and are highly wrought with volatile organic compounds (VOCs). Instead of buying the chemical laden leather polish, simply polish your shoes and leather goods with natural oil and a soft rag. Buying a cloth shower curtain ensures it's not emitting VOCs. Having your nails done is a common beauty regimen but there are healthier alternatives. Non-toxic nail polishes avoid five toxic elements—camphor, dibutyl phthalate (DBP), formaldehyde, formaldehyde resin, and toluene—linked to miscarriages, hormone imbalances, and cancer. Many cosmetic brands make non-toxic nail polishes that work just as well as the standard varieties, including topcoat. To remove the polish, use acetone. *Non-acetone solvents contain VOCs that contribute to air pollutants.* When buying any products with the potential for fumes, substitute for the non-VOC option.

Leather Polish

Olive or Vegetable Oil
Soft Rag

Apply oil liberally to the leather product with the rag. Allow to sit for 10 minutes to absorb. Buff to a shine with a dry soft cloth. For color shoe polish, add pigments that can be found online in their mineral form.

An alternative to aerosol sprays for automotive work is to drip jojoba oil with an eyedropper over the squeaky hinge or part. It is the most stable of natural alternatives and doesn't leave an unpleasant residue on the hinge, unlike other vegetable oils. For maximum coverage, give the door a swivel after applying the oil. Simply wipe off excess with a rag, as needed, and the door is as good as new. This all-natural alternative ensures you're not spraying potentially toxic chemicals in the house you eat, sleep, and breathe in.

Economical and Natural Recipes for Cleaning Solutions

Toxic aerosol disinfectants are commonly labeled with warnings not to inhale, get on skin, or spray near food, not only for their inherent toxic properties but, being volatile and airborne, they are also a source of VOCs in the home. Some disinfectants are linked to behavioral problems and chronic asthma in children, even when their exposure has been in utero. Super cleaners might accelerate superbug evolution when they kill 99.9% of germs, as claimed, making the survival of the 0.1% of remaining germs selected for reproduction. The recipes below are natural alternatives.

General Purpose Cleaner

1 Cup Water
1 Cup Vinegar

Combine in a spray bottle and use on all surfaces. This works great on all surfaces, including stainless steel appliances. Allow to soak for a minute, and wipe away with a clean rag.

Natural Disinfectant

1½ Cups Vinegar
1½ Cups Water
3 drops Lavender Essential Oil (Optional and Omit if Avoiding Plant Estrogen)

Combine in a spray bottle and shake before use on showers, toilets, and floors.

Tub and Tile Cleaner

½ Cup Baking Soda
¼ Cup Liquid Castile Soap
1-2 Tablespoons Water

In a small bowl combine to make a thick paste and gently scrub tub or shower floor with a sponge.

Toilet Bowl Cleaner

1 Cup Baking Soda
1 Cup Vinegar
1 Tablespoon Liquid Castile Soap

Combine everything in toilet bowl and scrub. Allow to sit for 10 minutes and flush.

Abrasive Deep Cleaner (for Barbecue Grill Grates or Baked-on Stains)

1 Cup Baking Soda
1 Cup Vinegar

Combine and apply liberally with gloved hands to the surface. Then cover the item so it's airtight. Allow to sit for 10-15 minutes then scrub with steel wool. Pieces of crumpled foil work just as well as steel wool in a pinch. Reshape and reuse the foil piece as needed.

Homemade Dish Soap

Ideally all dishes would be washed by hand to promote good immune development in children. Having your entire family help with after meal dishes establishes healthy routines and discipline, and is great for their overall health. Not washing dishes perfectly, as children might, actually leaves a residue of probiotics on the dishes and boosts immune health. Chores are also just an important life lesson. One day, when they are on their own, they'll be in the habit of helping. For convenience, here is a recipe for dish soap.

1 Cup Liquid Castile Soap
¼ Cup Water

Combine in a soap dispenser for easy hand and dish washing. An alternative is Castile bar soap. Combine 1 grated bar of soap with 3 cups of boiling water. Stir to combine and allow to cool before pouring into a soap dispenser.

Baking soda is a mainstay in natural cleaning. Keep a covered bowl of it in each place of cleaning: one in the bathroom, one in the kitchen, and one in the garage. Repurposing your old BPA plastic storage containers that cost a pretty penny back in the day fulfills one of the 3Rs of the green movement: Reduce, Reuse, Recycle. The cereal dispensers are especially handy for the toilet designated baking soda. Inexpensive liquid Castile soap is available online and at certain grocery stores. You can have some fun shopping around for Castile soap, with its differing scents, and take a look at the organic produce while you're at the store. Big box stores have large inexpensive bottles of vinegar and baking soda. Otherwise, they are easily available at the grocery store. The extra effort here is paid off by no contact with chemicals leaching into the air or skin, since many standard disinfectants are toxic to humans, can cause anxiety, and destabilize hormone balances.

Laundry and Stain Removal Tips

This recipe for laundry detergent was adapted after my cat developed skin allergies to standard detergents, prompting a quest for natural home alternatives for frequently used household items.

Homemade Laundry Detergent

1 Large Covered Container (2 Gallon Minimum)
1 Box of Washing Soda (55 oz.)
1 Box of Borax (65 oz.)
3 Bars of Castile Soap Finely Grated (4 oz. ea.)
1 Small Cup
1 Tablespoon Measure

The Castile soap may be grated like cheese, and with parental supervision kids can help with this part. A food processor with a fine grating attachment works well, too. Leave the rest of the steps to the adults and avoid contact with eyes or lungs because both borax and washing soda are caustic. Place everything in the container, and work outdoors in an open, ventilated area with a mask. Cover and toss the container for a few minutes until dry ingredients are well combined. Allow the dust to settle for five minutes before opening to use or dispense into other containers. Adding a scant 2 tablespoons to 4 tablespoons (¼ cup) per load of laundry will make this quantity last at least three months. Dissolve the mix in a small cup before adding to the machine. For HE-labeled (high efficiency) washing machines use a slightly mounded tablespoonful. Store in an airtight container.

For tough fabric stains, family-safe Castile soap bars are readily available in most supermarkets. Apply water to the stain before applying the bar directly and lathering. Give the stain a good dab with a damp cotton swab that has been smudged with Castile soap. For tougher fabrics, dampen the stain with water and scrub vigorously together with Castile soap. The sooner the stain has treatment the more likely it will be removed completely.

On tougher stains, enzymatic cleaner not only removes the stains pets leave behind but it also removes organic matter and stains from clothing. This cleaner is easily found online and is eco-friendly. Many standard stain removers are harmful to the environment with their petroleum-based ingredients. Apply liberally to the stain and allow to sit for one or two days for the enzymes to properly digest and degrade the organic matter. Keep in a spray bottle in a secure location around the house for easy application on stains on carpets or clothing.

Dryer Sheets

1 Old 100% Wool Sweater
Needle and thread
Scissors

Simply cut the sweater into pieces that will bundle into tennis ball size. Sew into a rough ball and throw into your dryer for permanent residence as a natural reducer of static electricity. Wool greatly reduces waste, since standard dryer sheets are made of wax-covered recycled paper that will end up being conveyed to landfills after one or two uses.

Also, clean up excess food scraps in the kitchen by composting food to avoid filling landfills with renewable resources. Rich soil is produced from compost comprising organic produce, paper towels, and food soiled paper goods. In a perfect world trash bins wouldn't exist and there would only be recycling and composting bins. Using green disposal bags and other biodegradable kitchen products for composting prevents adding mass to landfills. Corn based, disposable, single use utensils and food service products are mandatory in many cities and are a great way to limit your carbon footprint when you're away from home. Composting in organic home gardening teaches kids the lifecycle of food. It teaches environmental responsibility for air quality improvements from every plant grown.

Disposal of the toxic elements in your home might require some extra care. Make sure to take the extra step to talk to your local toxic or hazardous waste disposal site for information. Finding the extra time to do right by the earth is not only good for future generations, but teaches current generations sustainability.

By replacing harsh chemicals with organic and natural alternatives we can clean while prioritizing the health of our family and the Earth. The family-safe recipes and techniques are simple for the entire family to follow. We can help the world by cleaning without creating superbugs or contributing to health problems with harsh cleaners. Super cleaners exist for use in kitchens, bathrooms, and around the home, but it doesn't mean using them is better than natural cleaners. Knowing the damaging consequences of using harsh cleaners and making the switch to natural ensures a healthier family, home and planet. This is the beginning of an organic world. Live by example and others will follow.

Where We're Going

*Y*ou know what's best for you and your family, and it's okay if everything you've learned here doesn't resonate with you. The tips and tricks aren't meant to be the basis for a rigid routine or discipline, but are an alternative approach. When we start to change the way we see all inner workings of the home, we may see inconsistencies and anomalies we had never noticed before.

New possibilities of what it truly means to be eco-conscious is rewarding for us and for the future to discover. The more we delve into the nature of the chemicals that are commonly found in homes, the more opportunities we have for improvement. Companies behind these products can improve their formulas as not to contribute to superbug evolution nor harm us. We can also make choices not to purchase brands that have stances that are antagonistic to our newly discovered understandings. The good news is that countless companies are already making natural cleaning products.

Each small environmentally savvy change in caring for your health, home, and family will help you thrive and grow in this changing world. Your home and family will become more active, dynamic and energetic following a transition to natural cleaning products. You will notice fewer complaints of stomach pangs and digestive issues after the switch to some organic foods, along with increasingly healthy feelings. Food can be medicinal; in time your entire family will be radiant from wholesome alternatives to mass produced food. Don't forget to find time for yourself now and then. Self-appreciation shows others how to appreciate you! Enjoy the world! Stay Earth friendly!

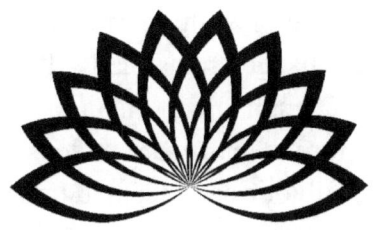

An Organic Future

*We do not inherit the Earth from our ancestors; we borrow it
from our children.*

—*Ancient Native American Proverb*

No matter where you are in your organic journey, healthy
living is possible because economical and organic recipes are
easily adaptable to any budget and time frame. Finding an extra
moment to assemble natural alternative recipes can be peaceful

and gratifying. Being creative, productive, and comfortable in all areas of your life can ease even seemingly stressful times. Living by example for your family and the betterment of society illuminates a beacon of health and kindness for all.

As increasing generations are born with an urgent desire to see the world in a greener, healthier, more peaceful state, how the world works will change dramatically. Plastic and chemical production becomes a laughable moment in history. Food additives that once were the norm are no longer mainstream. Mass injections of antibiotics are deemed unnecessary in food production as we gear towards lab grown meats. Slaughterhouses and large-scale animal farming are a distant memory. The greenhouse gas (methane), once overproduced in huge cattle lots, is reduced to record lows. Parasites, mad cow disease, and other transmittable ailments from food sources to humans are nonexistent. The oceans, once overfished, are bountiful and healthy once again as bans on all inhumane commercial fishing are enacted. Detailed descriptions on labels for all products is required, itemizing every active or inactive ingredient, chemical additives, and their potential interactions.

Farming practices must adapt to the banishment of toxic GMO crops, fertilizers, insecticides, and herbicides. Bees are healthy and abundantly vigorous again as they no longer are exposed to any neurotoxins in pesticides. Conscientious citizens might keep bee colonies in small hives as pets in their backyard, as well, giving Mother Nature a leg up. People know that attending to the well-being of all organisms in this world is just as important as for any family pet.

Trash and non-biodegradable objects are burned cleanly in government-run plants for generating green energy instead of ending up in landfills, our world's oceans, or waterways. Composting becomes the main means of treating household organic waste. Electric cars and trains eliminate one of the main historical sources of pollution. Fuel standards are applied to large ships, as they once burned the dirtiest fuels on the planet. Readily available and easily installable solar panels are so efficient they're even utilized in cities known for their perennial cloudy skies. The few gas run cars produced are fueled by biodiesel, probably used fry oil discarded by restaurants. Carbon producing goods have been reduced and all air conditioning units are now required to be eco-conscious. This main source for the warming of the lower atmosphere, in hot climates, is nonexistent and the atmosphere cools to record lows. Water quality is standardized as every home is retrofitted with lifelong filters and purifiers. Fracking is banned and all tainted water is no longer utilized. Rainwater is diverted automatically from gutters to water catchers for lawn and garden watering.

Most allergies and asthma are a thing of the past. Clean air quality standards coincide with the diminishing air pollution. Harsh chemicals that once irritated lungs of sensitive people have been identified and nixed from society. People live longer with ready access to organic food and proper clean water. Plastics are banned and the return to glass has its benefits since it is easy to upcycle, clean, and reuse without sending it back to the recycling plant. Washable, reusable, natural rubber bottle caps are common and there is a huge uptick in the market for old-fashioned milk caps. For commercial use, restaurants and food establishments store food in stainless steel and corn containers as alternatives for glass or plastic. All ready-to-eat foods are sold in improved corn based containers that hold contents for days instead of hours.

Down the food chain we see birds, amphibians, and other sensitive wildlife flourishing in places they once had abandoned or been driven away from by human encroachment. These organisms become plentiful again and are a positive beacon for change in the right direction. Waterways are no longer polluted with fertilizers and runoff from toxic gardening as these chemicals have been banned. Natural and organic farming practices have boosted the runs of salmon, tuna, trout, and other oceanic life from barren to abundant.

There is little waste because revitalizing Mother Nature has the top priority and takes precedence over either convenience or cost. Recycling is even cleaner than in the past and the incentives to recycle outweigh its added cost. In our globalized world, a common interest is the health of the planet. While some struggle with putting food on the table, it's up to other developed nations and societies to move the world towards a healthier and cleaner one. Setting up infrastructure is more important than monetary gain. Countries and societies deemed lost causes are a prime opportunity for the new world order to enact change and contribute extra services and supplies. This switch from corporate wars profiteering in foreign countries to societies helping one another and championing for change is possible. The opportunities are endless with the internet globalizing communication.

Instead of penalties for not following new rules, there is societal pressure to do what's right for the world. No longer is there need to police waterways for the dumping or spilling of toxic chemicals, as they are self-regulated. Proper action is always the priority and responsibility of the parties at hand without hesitation. The overall desire for everyone to have a clean, healthy world to live in outweighs any second-guessing of the right thing to do. It is ingrained in all members of society, in all parts of this globalized world. Every waste product from one industry is a raw material for use in another product, either recycled or repurposed. In all ways, the Earth heals and bounces back from the harm of past generations.

Eliminating toxic chemicals from all layers of society ensures a healthier world and future. The more efficient that societies become at maximizing their green potential, the more they can enjoy the world we live in. The future is bright in the generations that follow with their ideals for a better world. Being part of something that's bigger than oneself is a compelling dynamic for the future. We can all do our part today by taking care of what we have and how we live. Each purchase, consumption, or sale of a product has its environmental footprint. Are you doing your part to make a small daily change for a greener planet? If we all make just one move towards positivity even in our peace of mind, we will cumulatively make an immense difference.

But first, take care of yourself. You owe it to the world!

Bibliography

Adams, Mike. "Natural News Labs Publishes Heavy Metals Test Results For Seaweeds and Sea Vegetables: Kelp, Kombu, Wakame, Nori, Dulse and More." *Natural News.* 11 February 2014. Web. 6 June 2016. <http://www.naturalnews.com/043871_seaweeds_heavy_m etals_wakame.html>.

Angier, Natalie. "Animals and Fungi: Evolutionary Tie?" *The New York Times.* 16 April 1993. Web. 10 April 2016. <http://www.nytimes.com/1993/04/16/us/animals-and-fungi-evolutionary-tie.html>.

Appel, B R, J K Khalon, J Ferguson, et al. "Potential Lead Exposures from Lead Crystal Decanters." *American Journal on Public Health* 82(12) (1992): 1671-1673. *US National Library of Medicine: National Institutes of Health.* Web. 6 June 2016.

Atkinson, Fiona S., Kaye Foster-Powell, and Jennie C. Brand-Miller. "International Tables of Glycemic Index and Glycemic Load Values: 2008." *Diabetes Care* 3 October 2008: 2. PDF.

Burley, Gerard. "Read Your Labels." *Washington Blade.* 27 May 2016. Web. 6 June 2016. <http://www.washingtonblade.com/2016/05/27/read-your-labels/>.

Cohen, Michael H, Esq. "Web Disclaimer for Holistic Health Practice." *CAMLAW: Complementary and Alternative Medicine Law Blog.* 2015. Web. 4 February 2016.

<http://www.camlawblog.com/articles/general-business/web-disclaimer-for-holistic-health-practice/>.

Ehrlich, Steven D., NMD. "Turmeric." *University of Maryland Medical Center.* 26 June 2014. Web. 6 June 2016. <http://umm.edu/health/medical/altmed/herb/turmeric>.

Eilperin, Juliet. "Harmful Teflon Chemical To Be Eliminated by 2015." The Washington Post. 26 Jan. 2006. Web. 4 March 2016. <http://www.washingtonpost.com/wp-dyn/content/article/2006/01/25/AR2006012502041.html>.

Stein, Rob. "Kids, Allergies And A Possible Downside To Squeaky Clean Dishes." NPR. 23 Feb. 2015. Web. 4 March 2016. <http://www.npr.org/sections/health-shots/2015/02/23/387553285/kids-allergies-and-a-possible-downside-to-squeaky-clean-dishes>.

Graedon, Teresea and Joe Graedon. *People's Pharmacy: What's the best way to take aspirin for a heart attack.* The Seattle Times. 28 Oct. 2012. Web. 4 March 2016. <http://www.seattletimes.com/seattle-news/health/peoples-pharmacy-whats-the-best-way-to-take-aspirin-for-a-heart-attack/>.

Steinberger, Jillian. "The Future Strawberry: Will the Loss of a Major Pesticide Help the Industry to Go Green?" Civil Eats. 12 Jan. 2015. Web. 4 March 2016. <http://civileats.com/2015/01/12/the-future-strawberry-will-the-loss-of-a-major-pesticide-help-the-industry-to-go-green/>.

"Health Effects of Ozone in the General Population." *Environmental Protection Agency.* N.P., 22 Feb. 2016. Web. 4 Mar. 2016. <http://www3.epa.gov/apti/ozonehealth/population.html>.

Harris, Mark. "Why Consumers Are Buying Organic Spices." *E Magazine.* 8 May 2001. Web 4 March 2016.

<https://www.organicconsumers.org/old_articles/Organic/sp icesgood.php>.

Powell, Alvin. "The Entire Egg." *Harvard Gazette.* 24 Feb 2015. Web. 4 March 2016. <http://news.harvard.edu/gazette/story/2015/02/the-entire-egg/>.

Dahom, Gloria Gilbere. *Consumers Beware: Toxins Lurking in Your Clothing!* Total Health Magazine. 2011. Web. 4 March 2016. <http://www.totalhealthmagazine.com/Allergies-Asthma/Consumers-Beware-Toxins-Lurking-in-Your-Clothing.html>.

Harrington, Rebecca. *Does Artificial Food Coloring Contribute to ADHD In Children?* Scientific American. 27 April 2015. Web. 8 March 2016. <http://www.scientificamerican.com/article/does-artificial-food-coloring-contribute-to-adhd-in-children/>.

Hood, Ernie. "The Apple Bites Back: Claiming Old Orchards for Residential Development." *Environmental Health Perspectives* 114(8) (2006): A470-476. *Environews.* Web. 6 June 2016.

"How Much Arsenic Is in Your Rice?" *Consumer Reports.* 18 November 2014. Web. 6 June 2016. <http://www.consumerreports.org/cro/magazine/2015/01/how-much-arsenic-is-in-your-rice/index.htm>.

Kegley, S.E., B.R. Hill, and A. H. Choi. *PAN Pesticide Database. 2014. Web. 6 June 2016.* <http://www.pesticideinfo.org/Detail_Chemical.jsp?Rec_Id =PC35205>.

Kloc, Joe. "The Curious Case of the Chinese Chicken Import-Export Business." *Newsweek: Tech & Science.* Web. 6 June 2016. <http://www.newsweek.com/2014/10/10/curious-case-chinese-chicken-import-export-business-273699.html>.

Lehrer, Jennifer K., MD. "Food Labeling." *Medicine Plus*. U.S. National Library of Medicine. 15 May 2014. Web. 6 June 2016. <https://www.nlm.nih.gov/medlineplus/ency/article/002459.htm>.

Lorenzen, Janne Kunchel, Sanne Nielsen, Jens Juul Holst, et al. "Effect of Dairy Calcium or Supplementary Calcium Intake on Postprandial Fat metabolism, Appetite, and Subsequent Energy Intake." *American Society for Clinical Nutrition* 85 (2007):678-687. *Nutrution.org*. Web. 6 June 2016.

"Much High Fructose Corn Syrup Contaminated With Mercury, New Study Finds." *Institute for Agriculture and Trade Policy*. 26 January 2009. Web. 6 June 2016. <http://www.iatp.org/documents/much-high-fructose-corn-syrup-contaminated-with-mercury-new-study-finds>.

Rice, Hannah. "Advances in Human Microbiome Science: Gut-Brain Interaction." *The New York Academy of Sciences*. 26 May 2016. Web. 6 June 2016. <http://www.nyas.org/Publications/Ebriefings/Detail.aspx?cid=f215e92d-82e3-45cf-a10a-e8c3f669b10e>.

Stevens, William K. "Long Line Fishing Seen as Damaging to Some Fish and to the Albatross." *The New York Times*. 5 November 1996. Web. 6 June 2016. <http://www.nytimes.com/1996/11/05/science/long-line-fishing-seen-as-damaging-to-some-fish-and-to-the-albatross.html?pagewanted=all>.

Tucker, Johnathon, Ph.D. "Agricultural Biotechnology; Safety, Security, and Ethical Dimensions: Genetically Modified crops." *Federation of American Scientists*. Web. 6 June 2016. <http://fas.org/biosecurity/education/dualuse-agriculture/2.-agricultural-biotechnology/genetically-engineered-crops.html>.

Vien, Anya. "More Than Just a Condiment? Unbelievable Health Benefits of Mustard." *LA Healthy Living.* 26 September 2013. Web. 6 June 2016.

Walker, Bill. *Chemicals In Food Wrappers And Outdoor Clothing Linked To Spike In Miscarriages.* Enviroblog. 4 May 2015. Web. 8 March 2016. <http://www.ewg.org/enviroblog/2015/05/chemicals-food-wrappers-and-outdoor-clothing-linked-spike-miscarriages>.

Walton. Alice G. "Cash Register Receipts May Be A Source of BPA, Study Suggests." *Forbes.* 22 October 2014. Web. 6 June 2016. <http://www.forbes.com/sites/alicegwalton/2014/10/22/cash-register-receipts-may-be-a-source-of-bpa-study-suggests/#34632da01fbb>.

About the Author

Flora Jade has always known her purpose, and strives for a better world. Like many eco-conscious souls, she prides herself on her nature-oriented background from growing up in the Pacific Northwest. Please visit her website www.theflorajade.com for up-to-date blog posts and information about her new work.

We hope you enjoyed this Organic Publishing House book. If you'd like to receive more information please visit our website:

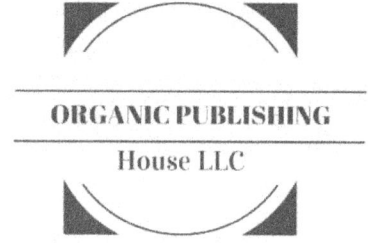

www.organicpublishinghouse.org

www.ingramcontent.com/pod-product-compliance
Lightning Source LLC
Chambersburg PA
CBHW060338290526
45793CB00003B/653